THE
40 MOST AMAZING
FARMS
IN THE WORLD

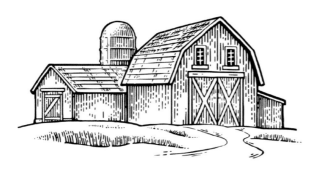

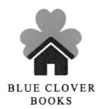

BLUE CLOVER
BOOKS

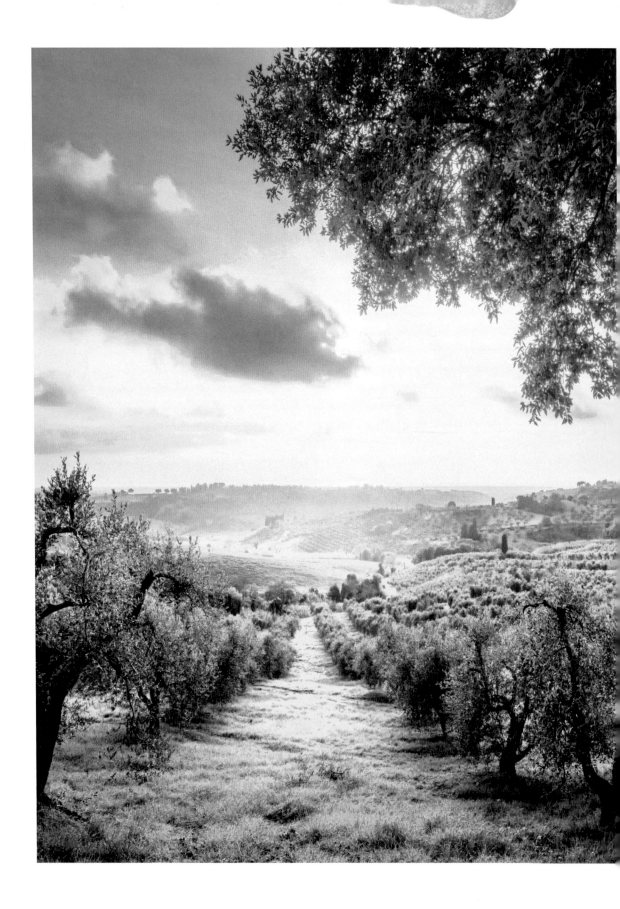

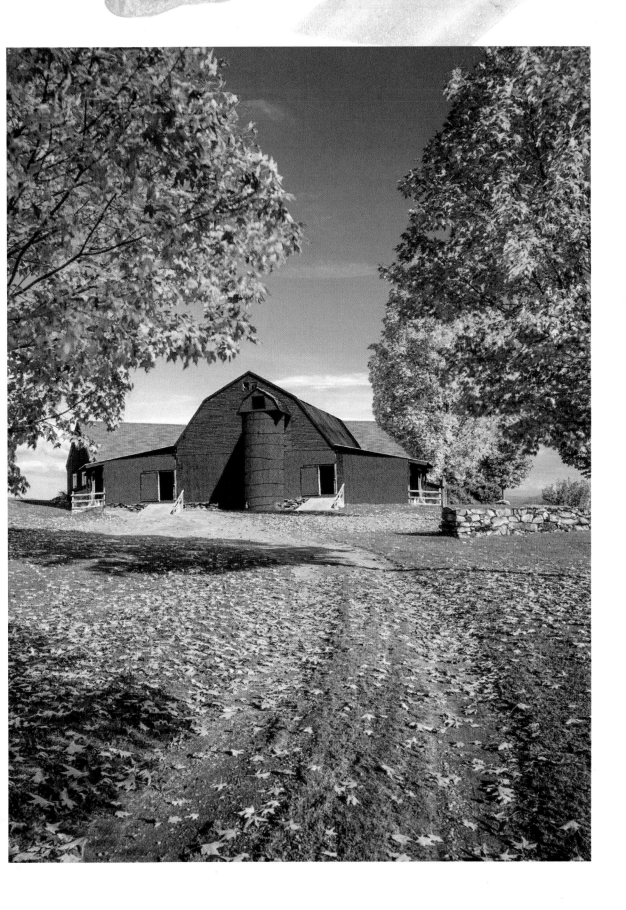

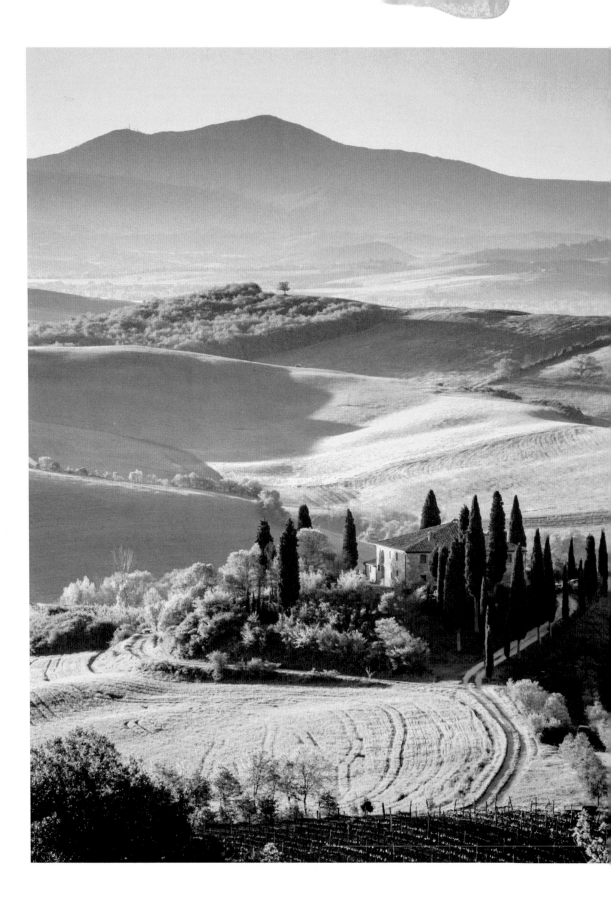

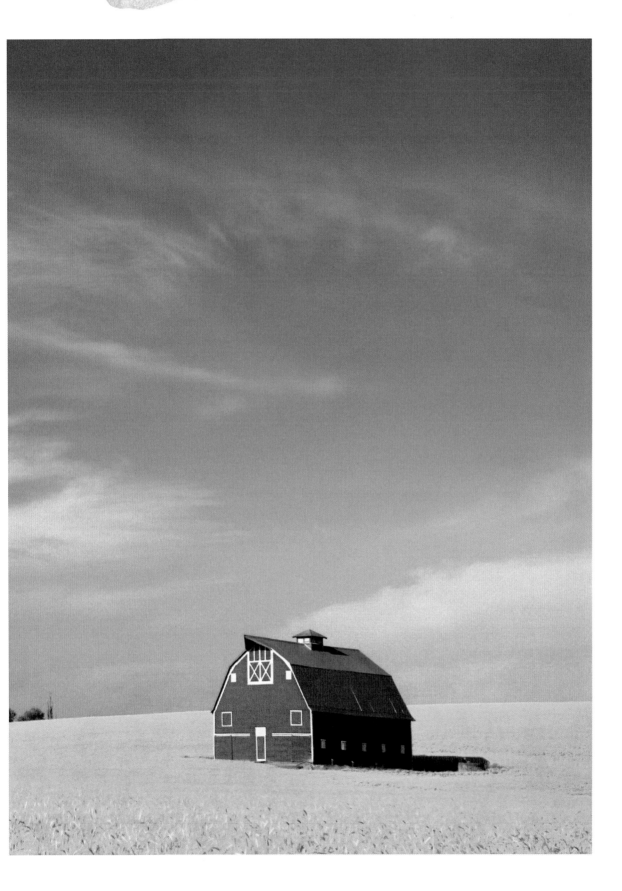

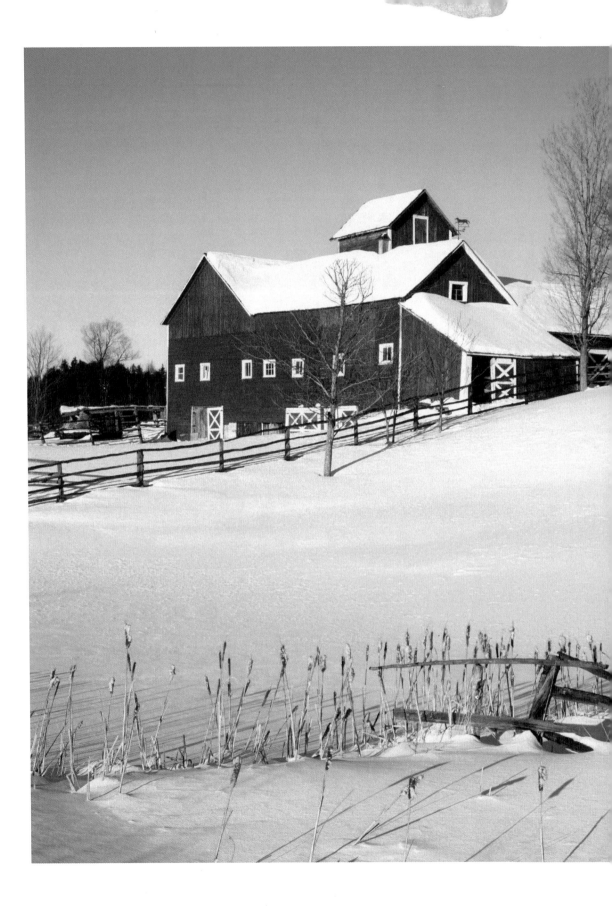

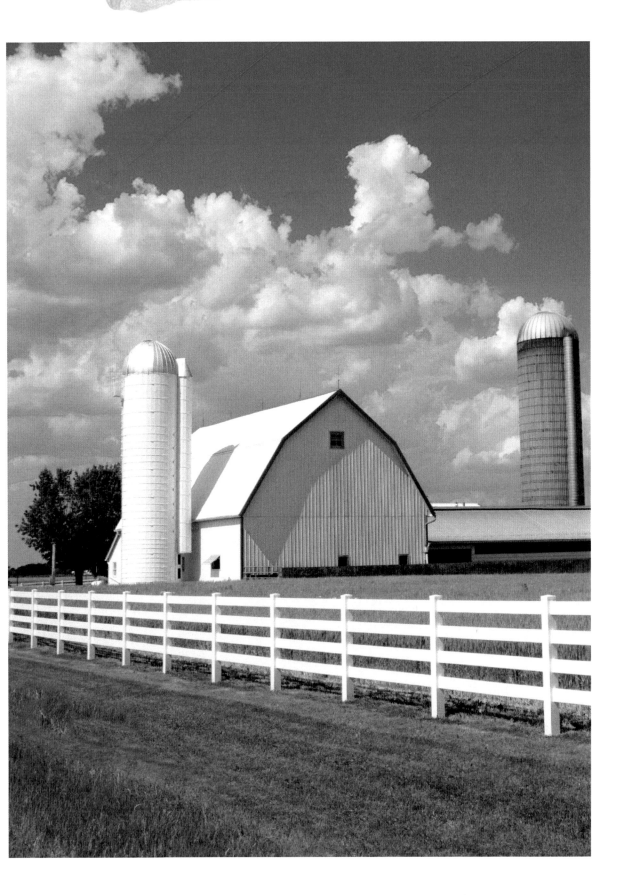

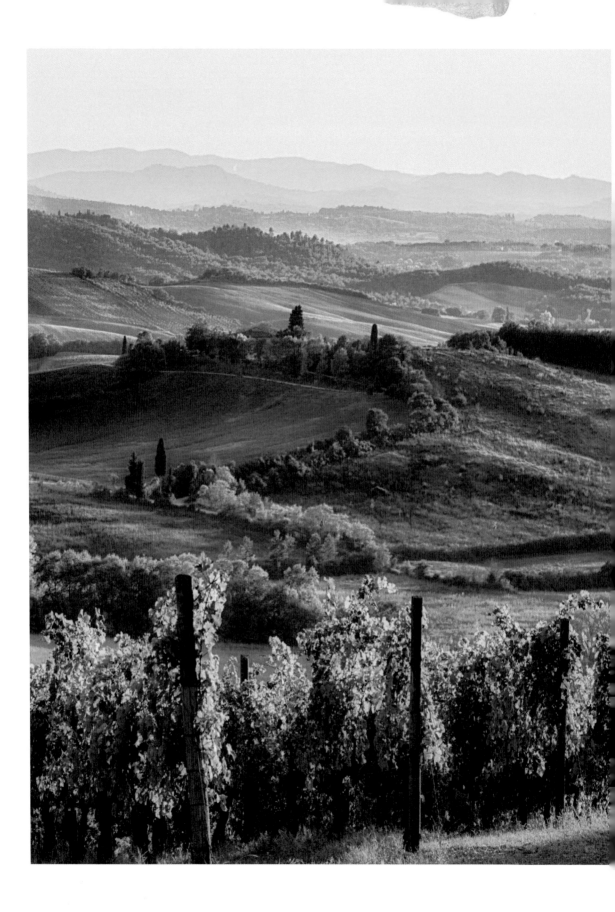

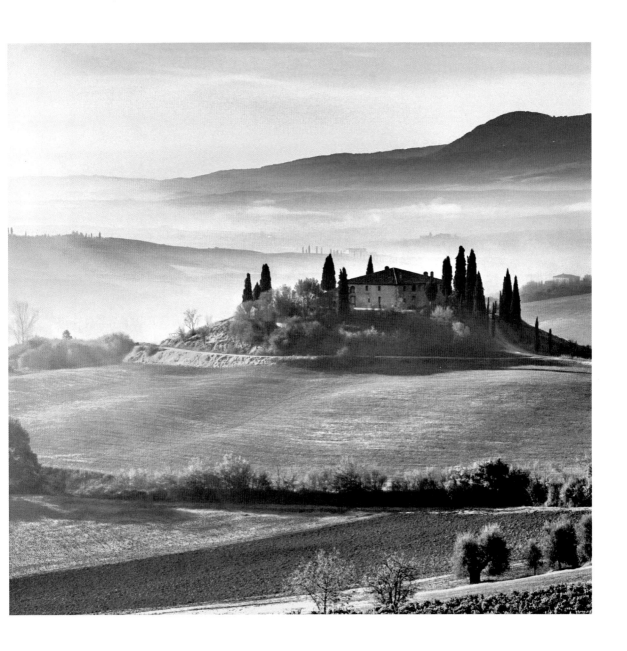

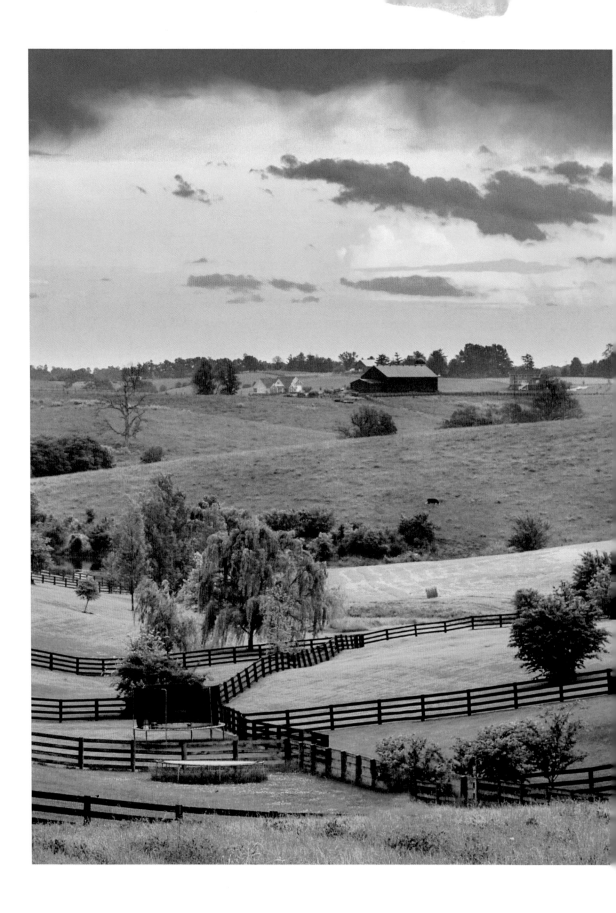

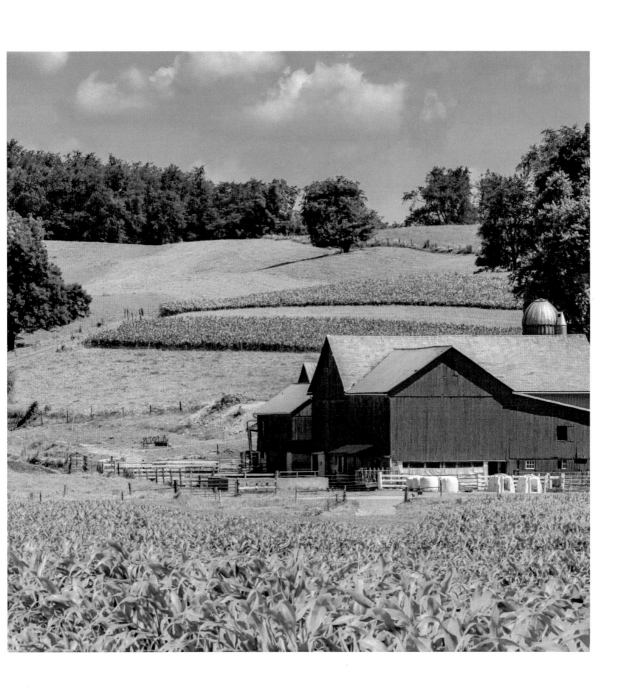

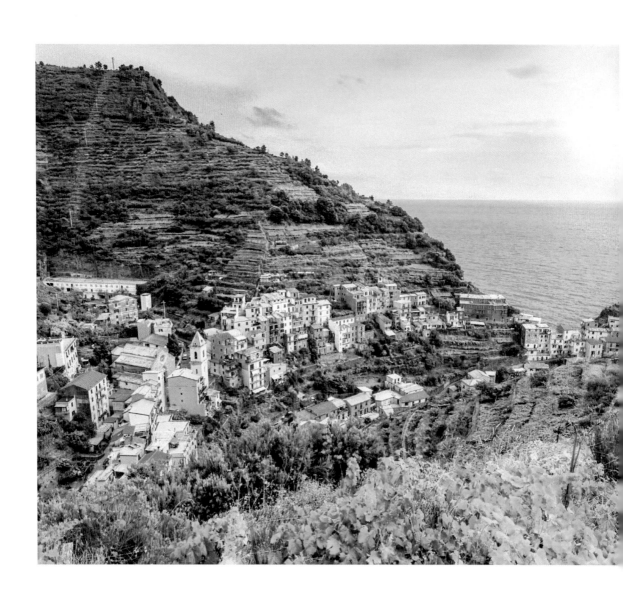

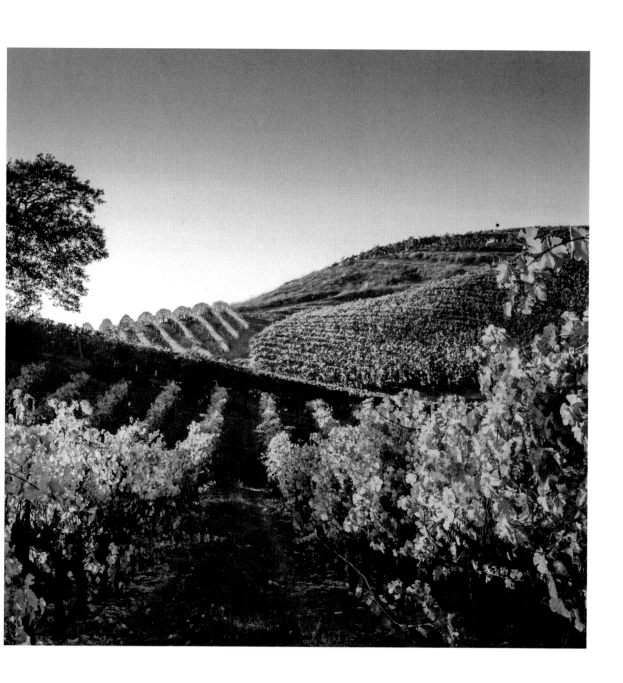

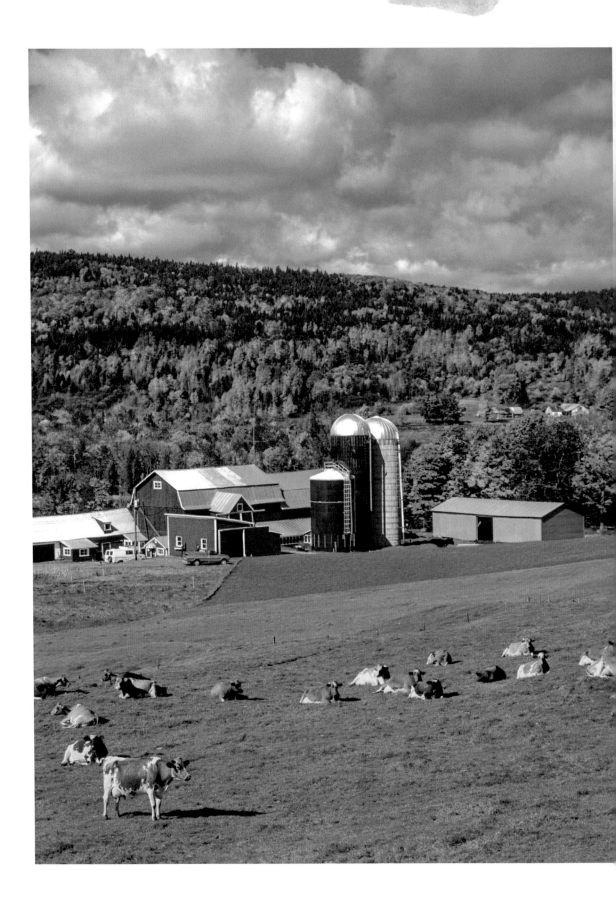

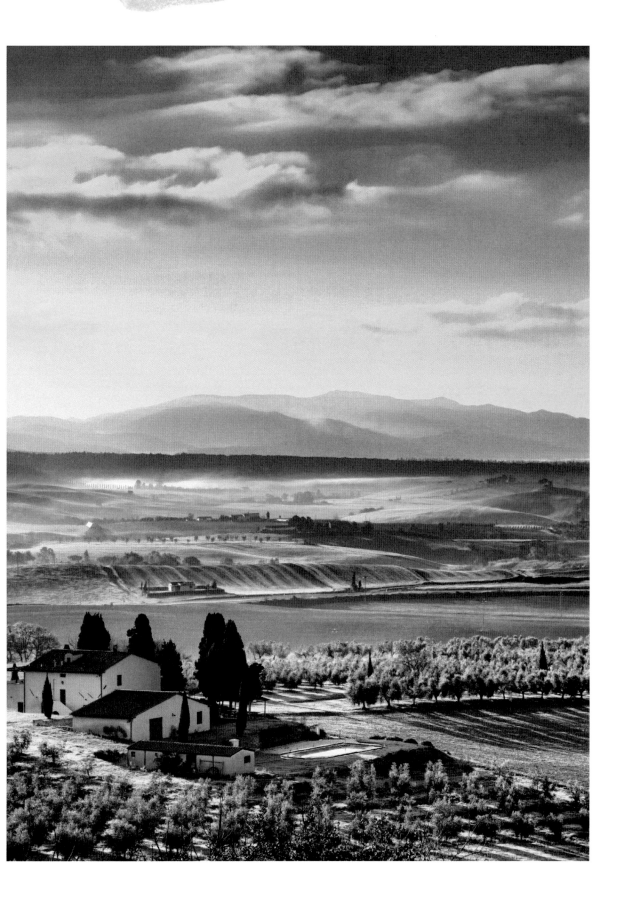

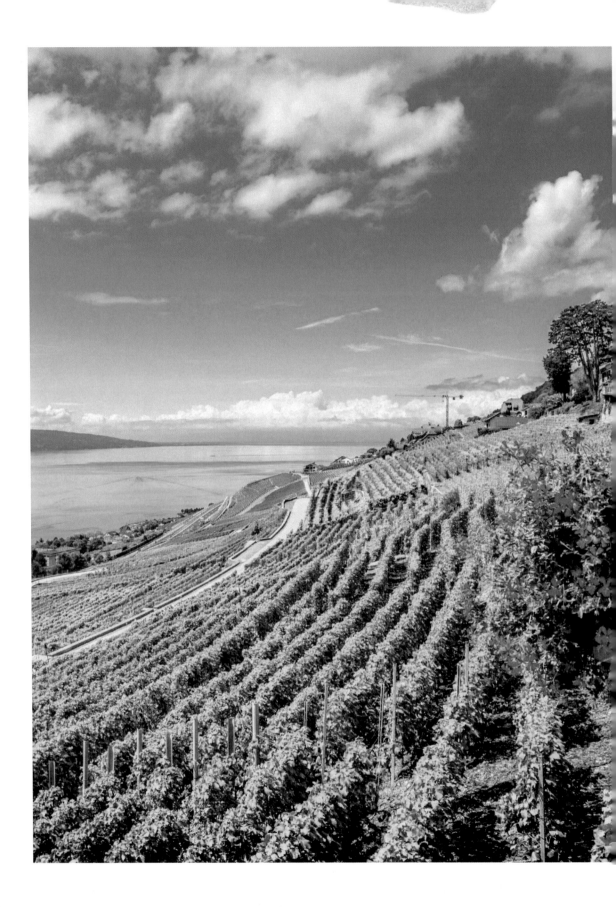

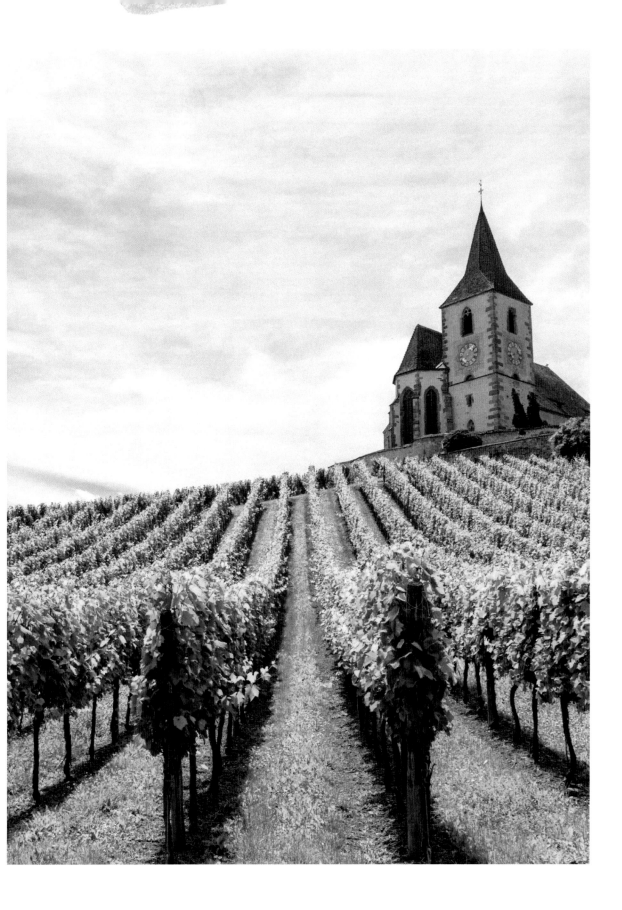

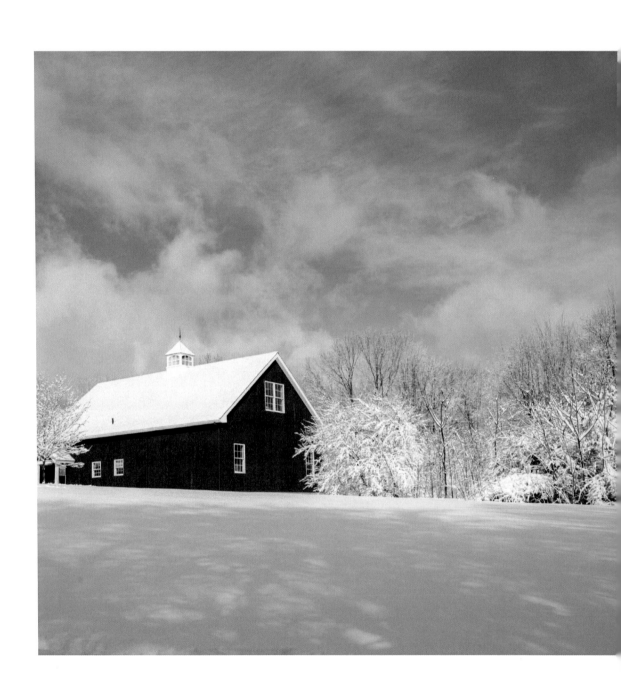

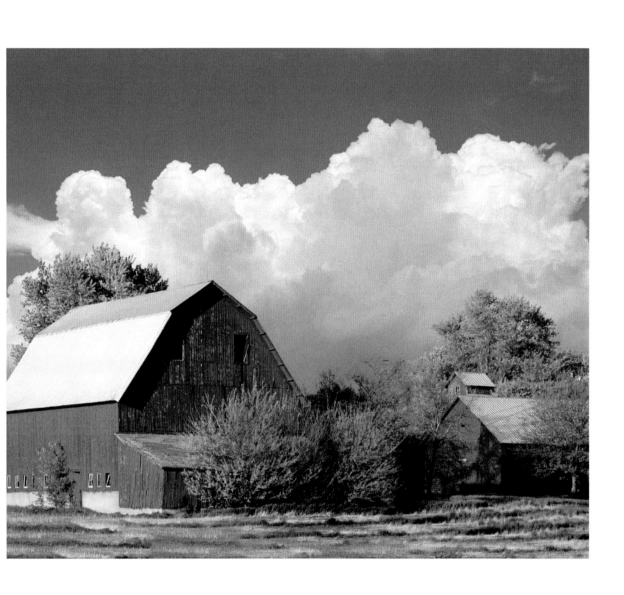

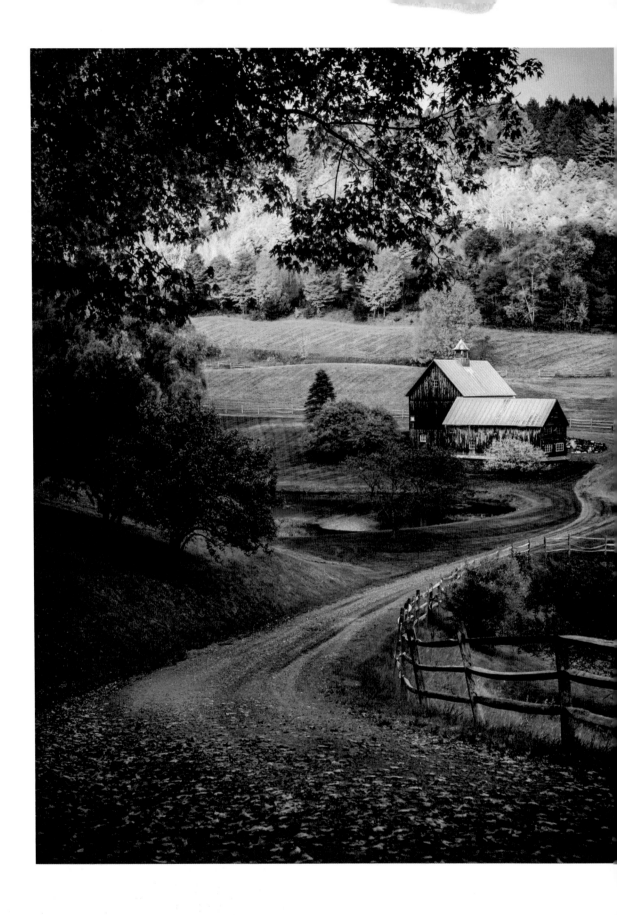

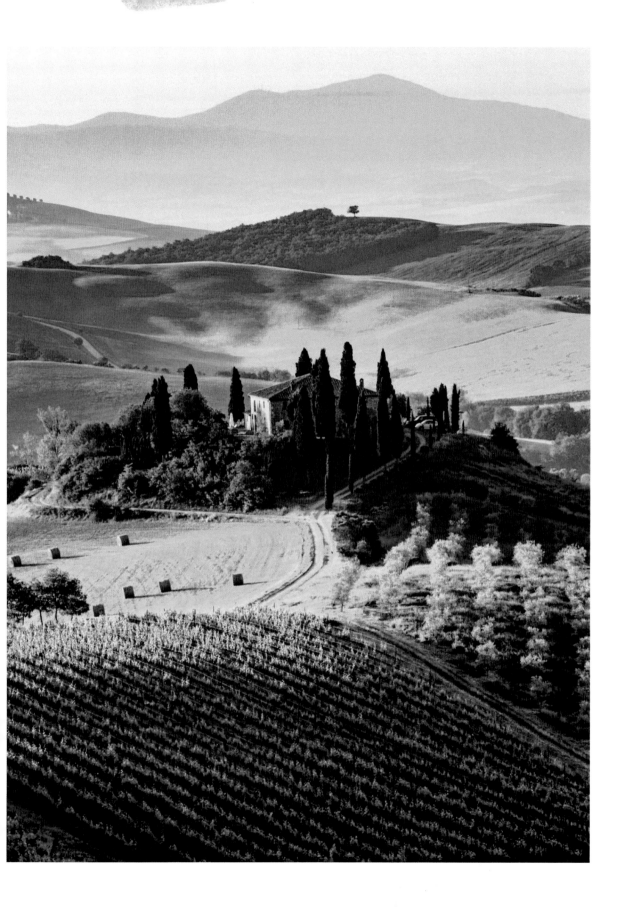

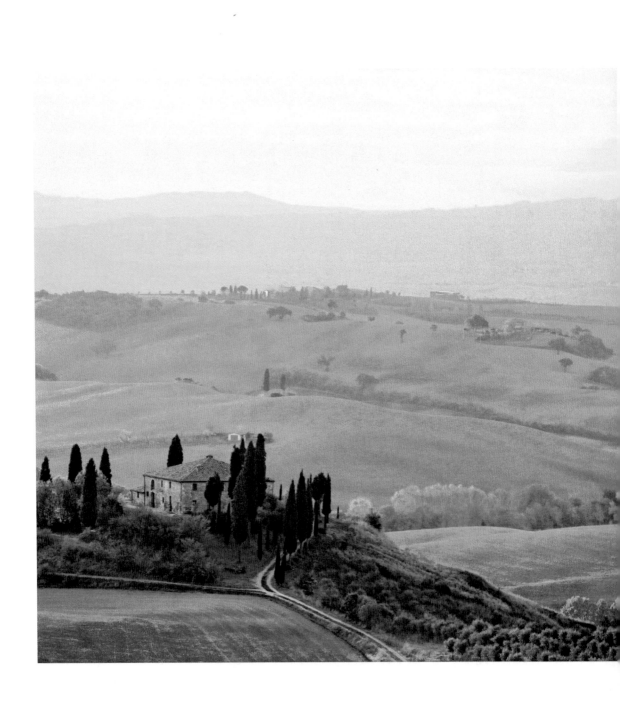

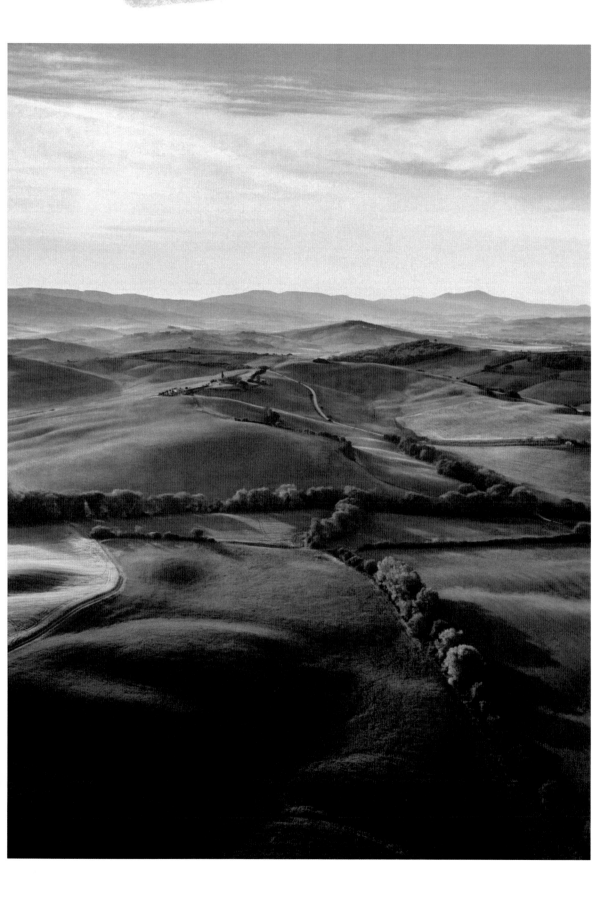

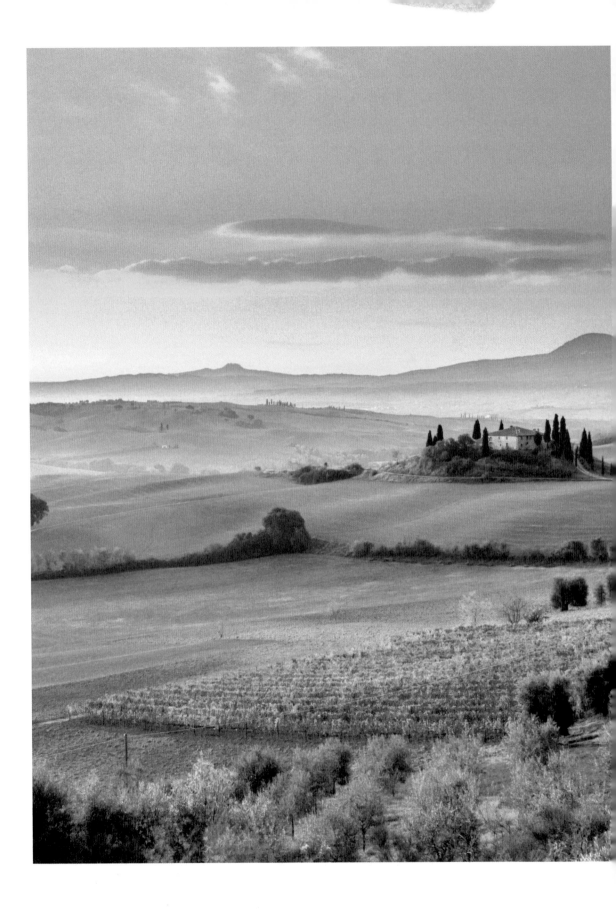

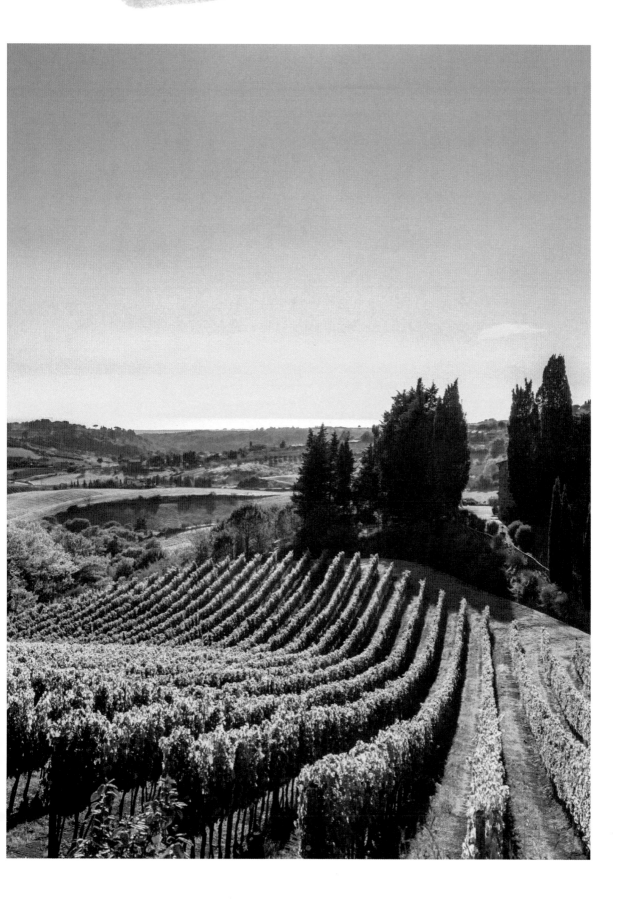

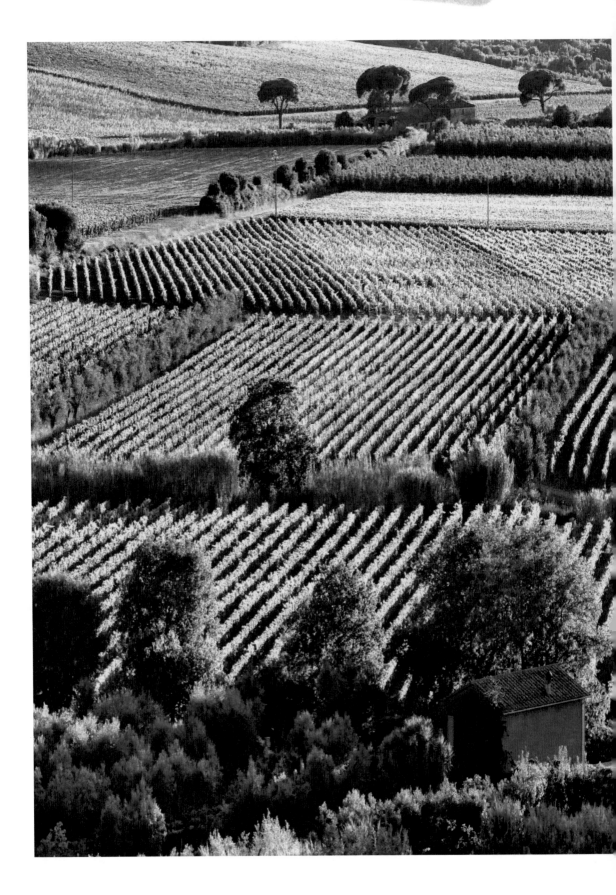

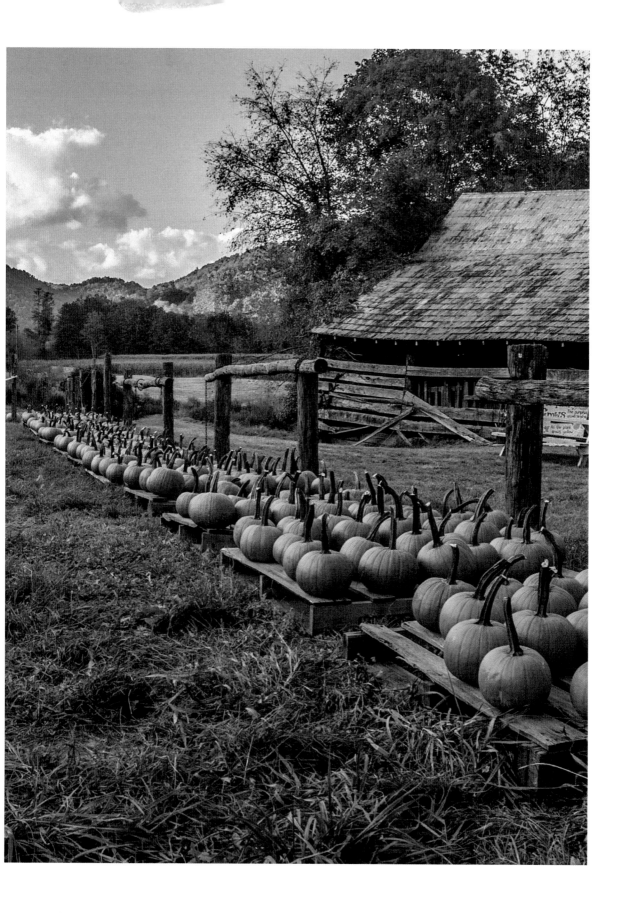

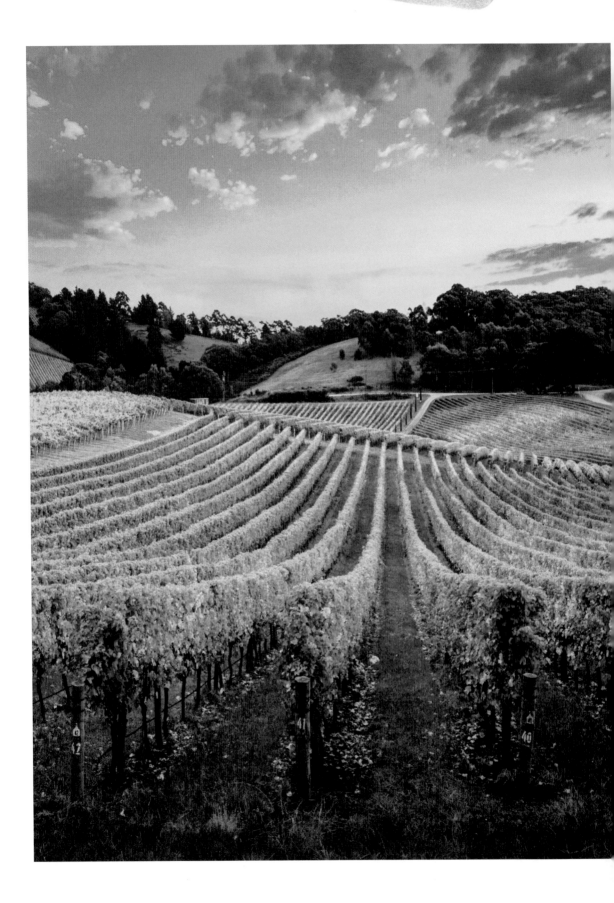

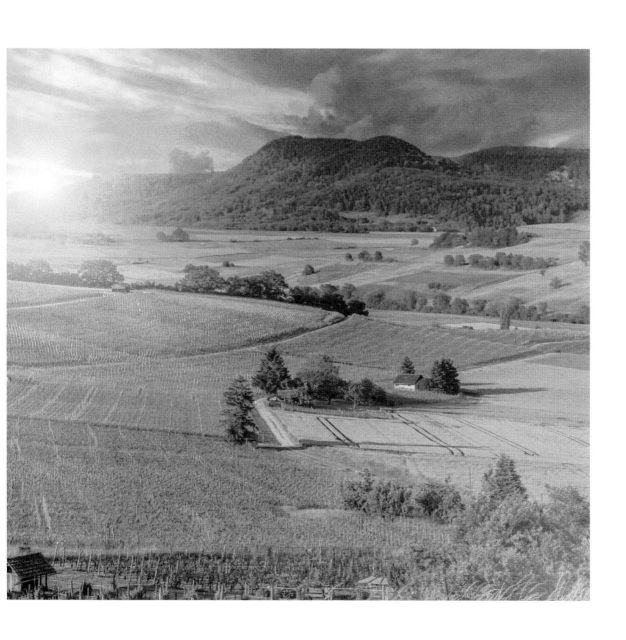

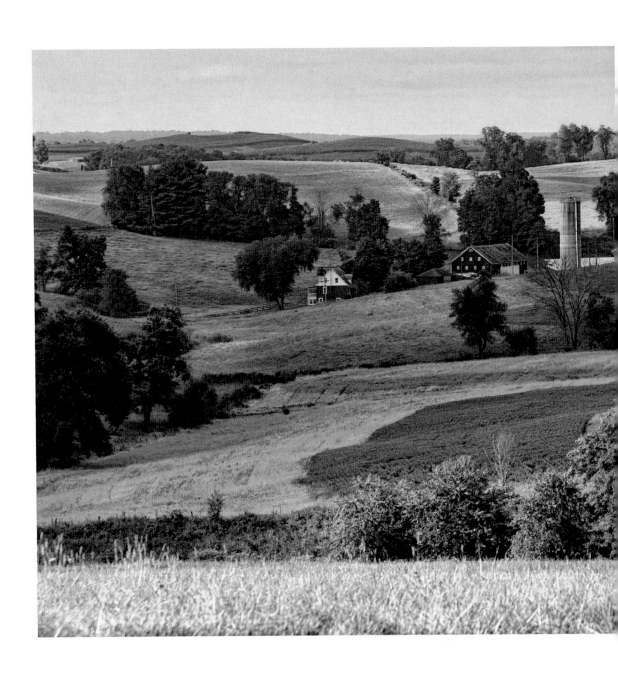

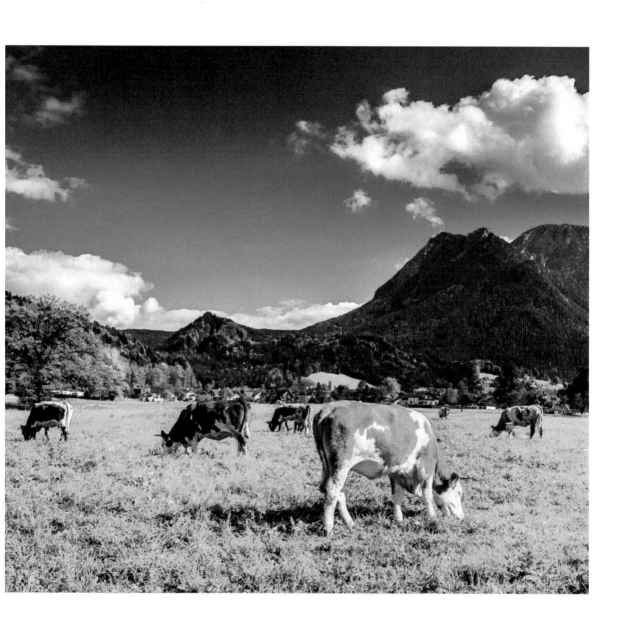

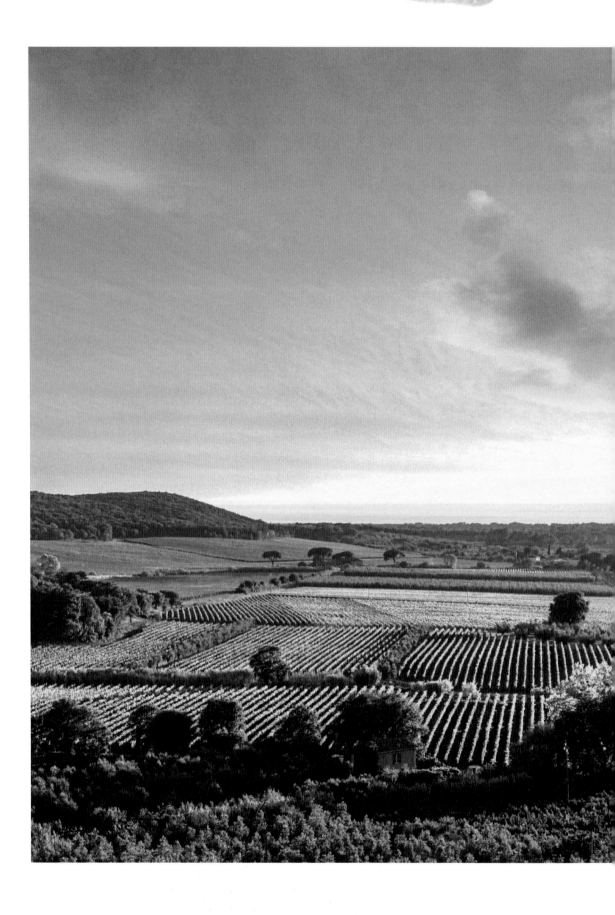

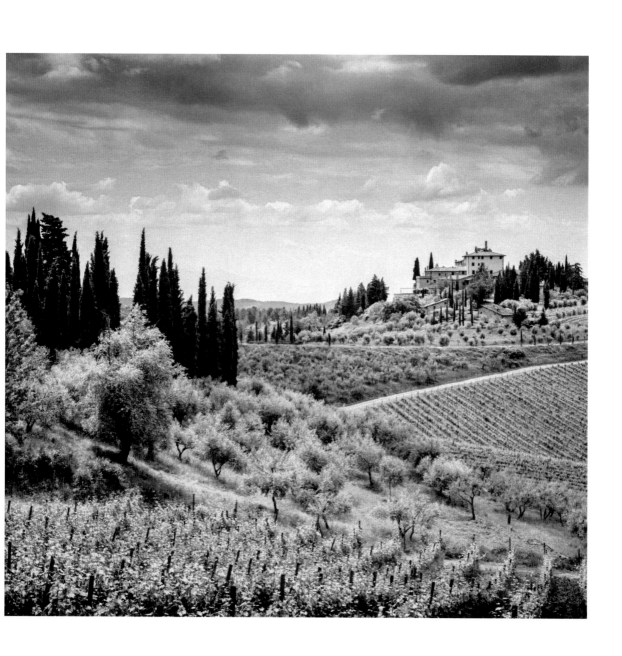

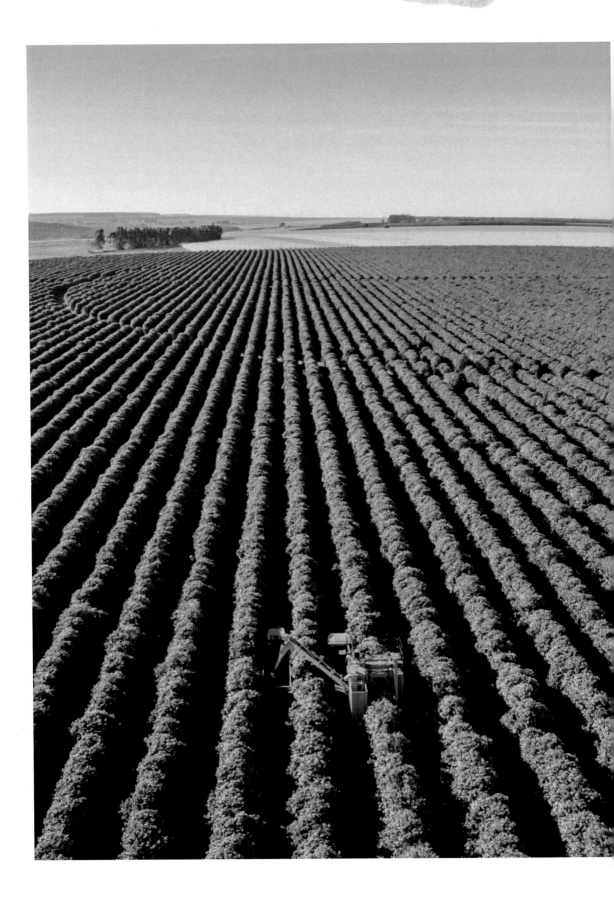

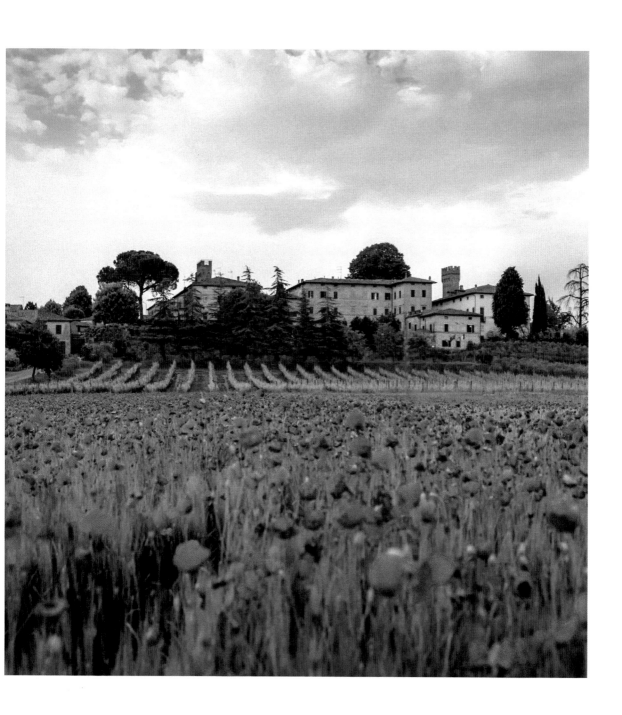

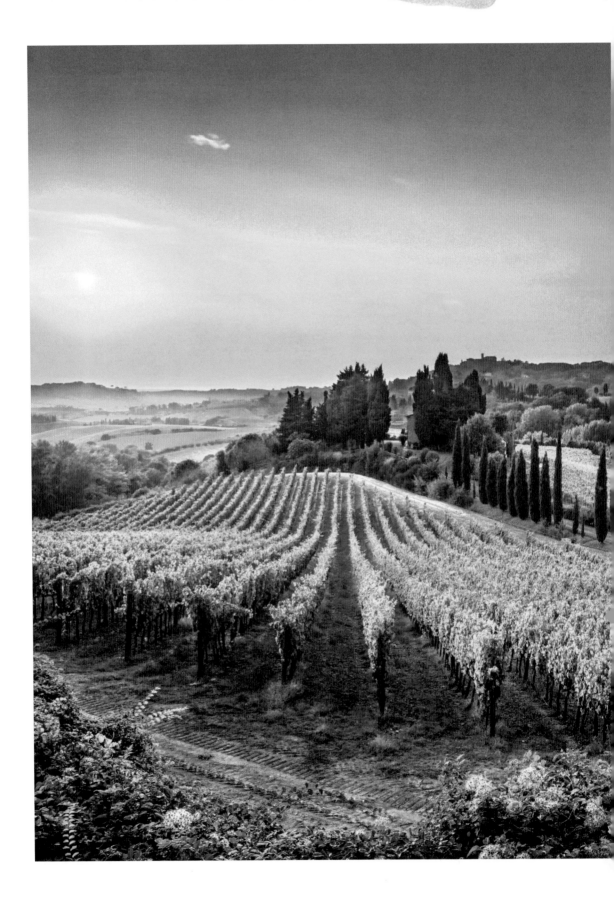

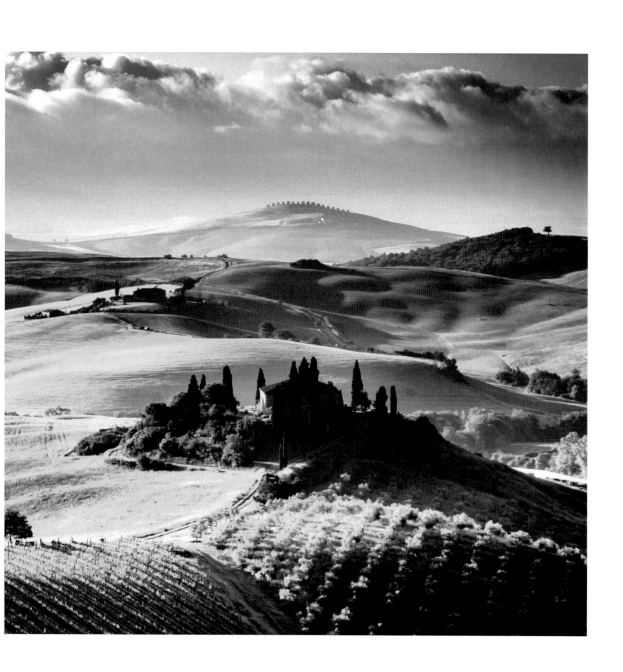

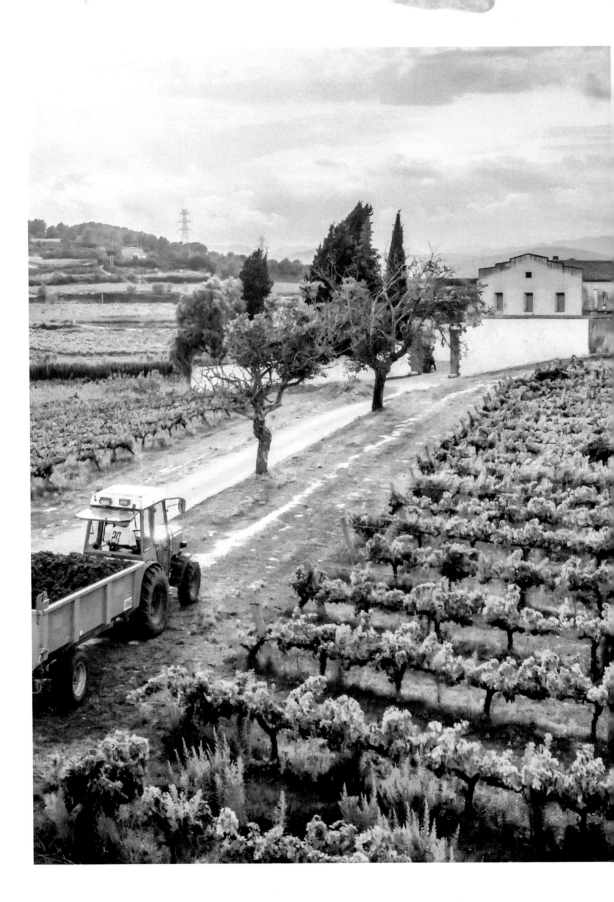

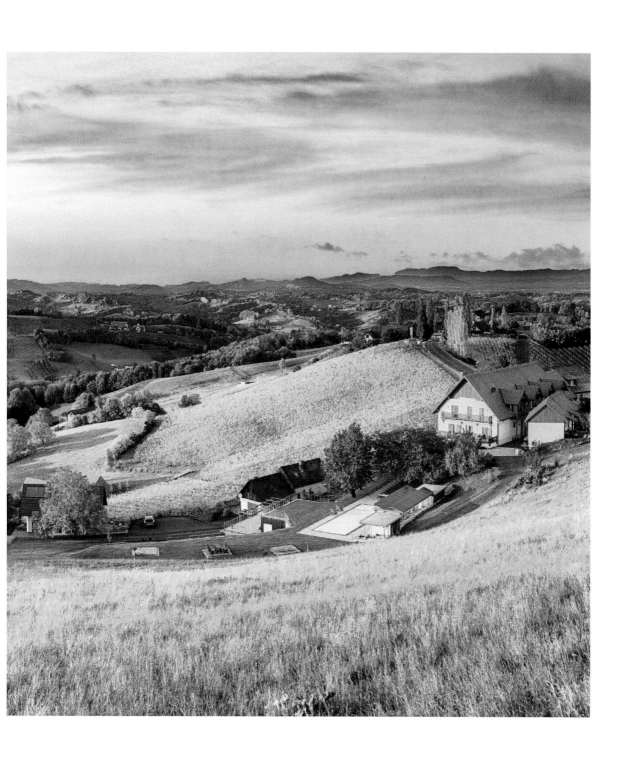

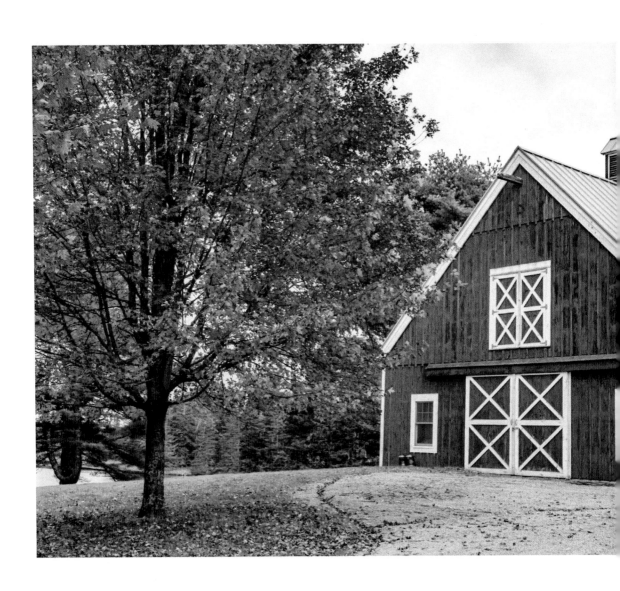

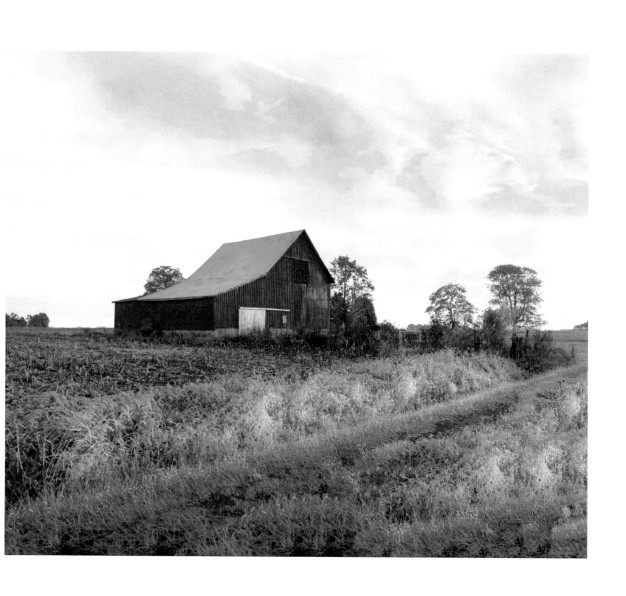

Thank you

Thanks for your interest in our books.

Please consider purchasing our other books
available now at Amazon.com.

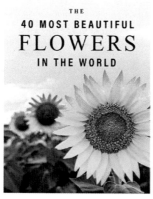
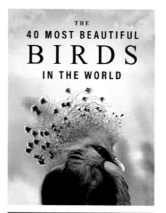
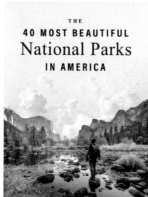
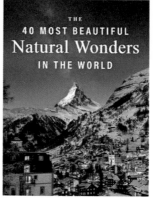

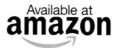
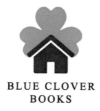

Made in United States
Orlando, FL
16 September 2024

51606296R00024